GROWTH MINDSET

MINDSET

THE UNSTOPPABLE YOU

MARCUS JOHANSSEN

D1518682

CONTENTS

To all those hoping to improve their lives, this book is dedicated to you. May it inspire you to embrace a growth mindset and cultivate the courage to turn your aspirations into reality. Remember, your greatest limitations are not what you can't do, but what you believe you can't do. So believe in yourself, trust the journey, and never stop growing.

INTRODUCTION

"It's kind of fun to do the impossible." This quote from Walt Disney perfectly embodies his belief that tackling difficult and seemingly impossible tasks can be both enjoyable and rewarding. Starting out as a simple cartoonist, Disney worked tirelessly to build his legacy and create one of the most iconic and successful entertainment companies in the world. But how did he do it? Was it just luck or was it his mindset that made the difference?

Disney was no stranger to challenges throughout his career. Financial struggles, intellectual property disputes, technological limitations, harsh critics, and fierce competition, all were obstacles he had to overcome. But instead of giving up, he persevered and pushed forward with enthusiasm. He didn't let the difficulties stop him from achieving his dreams, and this unwavering determination can be attributed to his growth mindset. He believed that with hard work and perseverance, he could achieve anything he set his mind to.

He not only believed in the power of hard work and perseverance, but he lived by it. He was a true inspiration, showing us that with a growth mindset, anything is possible.

So what is a growth mindset? It is the belief that with effort, learning, and persistence, you can continuously improve and develop your abilities and intelligence. Through it, you can create a world where your true potential is unlocked and nothing is hindering you from going after your dreams.

On the opposite side of the spectrum is the fixed mindset, which promotes limiting beliefs that hold you back. It tells you that your abilities and intelligence are set in stone, and you can't change them.

A growth mindset and a fixed mindset can be easily illustrated in how an individual approaches a difficult math problem.

If an individual has a growth mindset, they would view this problem as an opportunity to learn and grow. They would embrace the challenge and spend a significant amount of time trying to understand the problem, breaking it down into smaller parts, and figuring out different ways to solve it. They would not be discouraged by the difficulty of the problem and would be willing to take the time to learn from their mistakes. They would also be open to feedback and suggestions, using them as a learning tool to improve their understanding of the problem.

On the other hand, an individual with a fixed mindset would approach the problem differently. They would see the problem as a threat to their intelligence and might give up quickly if it seems too difficult. They would be less likely to put in the effort to understand the problem and might avoid it altogether. They would also be less open to feedback and less willing to learn from their mistakes. They would be more focused on proving their intelligence and abilities rather than improving them.

The approach to problem-solving and learning is vastly different between the two. One encourages an individual to embrace challenges, learn from mistakes and continuously improve, while the other limits the individual's potential and hinders their ability to learn and grow.

Why is it so important for you to embrace a growth mindset?

First and foremost, it will lead to increased resilience. Resilience is the ability to bounce back from setbacks, adapt to changes, and handle difficult situations with grace and determination. People with resilience tend to view challenges and failures as opportunities for learning and growth, rather than as setbacks or defeats. This ability to bounce back from setbacks more easily can help individuals to achieve their goals and overcome obstacles.

Second, it can change the way you think about stress and anxiety and learn to manage it in a healthier, more productive way. Learnign to do this successfully will have a positive influence on your physical health, cognitive function, and emotional well-being.

Third, it will lead to better self-esteem. When individuals understand that their abilities and intelligence can be developed, they tend to have a more positive self-image. They don't see themselves as limited by their current abilities, but rather as capable of growth and improvement.

Fourth, it will lead to a greater ability to adapt. Those who are open to new experiences and ideas are more resilient when things don't go as planned. They understand that the world is constantly changing, and they are better equipped to navigate these changes and come out on top.

In a word, the importance of a growth mindset lies in the fact that it can lead to greater success and well-being in all areas of life. It can help individuals to reach their full potential and achieve their goals by providing them with the tools they need to overcome challenges, learn from failures and grow. Embracing such a powerful tool is an important step towards a more fulfilling and successful life.

In this book, we're going to explore the absolute BEST ways to cultivate a growth mindset. As we do, we ask that you fully embrace not only the information being presented but the activities that take place along the way. Each of these interactive activities is designed to help you cultivate and manifest this mindset in real-time and will have a massive, positive impact on your mindset now and into the future.

So, let's get right into it with the first step, embracing discomfort.

CHAPTER ONE: EMBRACE DISCOMFORT

"Discomfort is the currency of your dreams."
- Brooke Castillo (Founder and CEO of The
Life Coach School)

WHAT IF I TOLD you that being uncomfortable was the key to success, would you believe me? One of the most dangerous places anyone could ever find themselves is their own comfort zone. Doing the things they've always done, eating the things they've always eaten, watching the things they've always watched, feeling the way they always feel, making the excuses they always make.

As humans, a huge part of our lives is spent in our comfort zone because it's easy to stay there, even if it isn't beneficial. Think about this in terms of your daily routine.

Which hand do you use to brush your teeth? Whichever hand it is, I guarantee it's the same hand you use every day. When you take shower in what order do you wash? Whichever order it is, I can guarantee it's the same order as it is every day. When you go to sleep at night, which side of the bed do you sleep on? Whichever side it is, I guarantee it's the same that you go to sleep on every night. When you put your socks on, which foot do you put them on first? I guarantee it's the same for that you always start with.

You do all of this because it makes life easier or more "comfortable." Let's make no mistake, just because it's easier or comfortable does not mean its good for you or fills you with positive feelings and motivation, it's just easier.

So, if you wanted to change the hand you brush your teeth with, what would you have to do? You'd have to think about changing it. Once you act upon that thought, that, in turn, would create new feelings and experiences. Some of those feelings are going to be uncomfortable, but this is the key to growth and self-improvement.

There's a fantastic story about the lobster and the process of shedding its shell. A lobster has a rigid shell that protects it and makes it feel safe. As it grows, it becomes too big for its shell and it starts to feel cramped and uncomfortable. The lobster begins to realize that its rigid shell is no longer serving its purpose and that it needs to shed it in order to grow and thrive.

The lobster is hesitant to shed its shell because it's familiar and it feels safe. But eventually, it realizes that it must let go of its old shell in order to grow and expand. The process of shedding its shell is uncomfortable and it takes time, but once it's done, the lobster is able to move and explore more freely.

This story is a metaphor for human life. We often become attached to our own rigid shells, whether it's our beliefs, habits, or routines. These shells can provide a sense of security, but they can also limit our growth and potential. Like the lobster, we need to be willing to shed our old shells and embrace change in order to grow and thrive. The process may be uncomfortable and take time, but it's necessary for our personal and professional growth. So, don't be afraid to let go of what no longer serves you and embrace change, you'll be surprised at what you're capable of.

In order to bring us into a positive state of welcoming change and discomfort, I'd like you to start thinking about some personal goals of yours. By goals, we're talking about a desired result that you would like to achieve. Here are a few examples of what a goal could sound like:

- I would like to be more punctual for work and other planned engagements.

- I would like to lose a couple of inches around my waist.

- I would like to improve my social skills.

- I would like to improve my study habits.

I'd like you to spend a few minutes thinking about some personal goals of yours, and when you're done, write down 1-3 things that come to mind.

1)

2)

3)

In self-help books and seminars, you'll often hear things like "massive change for massive success," or "take drastic action now." If that works for you, great. But I'd like to present another concept to you that in many ways is more manageable, and that's the concept of marginal gains.

The concept of "marginal gains" refers to the idea of making small, incremental improvements in various areas of a process or system in order to achieve a significant overall improvement.

With this concept is the amazing story of the British cycling team. Before the implementation of the marginal gains approach, the British cycling team had limited success in major international competitions. The team had not won a gold medal in the Olympic Games or the Tour de France, which are considered to be the two most prestigious events in the sport of cycling. The team, led by Dave Brailsford, applied the principle of marginal gains to many areas of their training and performance. Some examples of the specific gains they pursued include:

- Improving the fit of their clothing and equipment, to reduce drag and increase comfort.

- Washing hands frequently to avoid infection and sickness that would impact their performance.

- Paying attention to their diet, sleep, and recovery to ensure optimal performance.

- Providing the riders with the most comfortable mattress and pillows to promote good sleep.

- Using different types of massage and other therapies to speed up recovery.

- Providing the team with the best possible weather forecast to plan training and racing schedule.

The point is to find ways to improve by 1% in certain areas, the sum of all these small improvements will lead to a significant overall improvement in performance. Now let's make no mistake, just because it is a marginal gain doesn't mean there won't be discomfort or that it will be easy to achieve, this will still require effort and consistency. However, what it does mean is that achieving your goals or desired results will be more manageable.

Now let's get back to your personal goals.

Let's say one of your goals was to lose a few inches around your waist. Applying the theory of marginal gains, instead of going on a crash diet, you would begin by identifying small changes to your dieting or exercise habits that will help you achieve that goal. For example, if you like to eat ice cream in the evenings, you might start by reducing the portion size from 1 cup to 3/4 of a cup each time you have a bowl. After a week, you can reassess and see if there is room for further reduction or if another small change can be made, such as incorporating more fruits and vegetables into your diet, or a few minutes of cardiovascular exercise each day. Once again, although this is a small change, it will require consistency and working through a measure of discomfort, but with that discomfort will come positive growth.

Take another scenario for example. Maybe you would like to improve your social skills. Instead of avoiding social situations or making excuses not to socialize with others, start by setting a marginal gain of engaging in a social activity once a month. This can be as simple as going to a friend's house for a small gathering or inviting some coworkers out for a meal. As you become more comfortable, you can gradually increase the frequency of these activities. Remember, the discomfort you feel during the process will lead to growth.

You see, avoiding the thing that makes you uncomfortable is reinforcing the patterns, thoughts, beliefs, attitudes, and behaviors that you've been displaying. Real change means making change happen, and implementing the theory of marginal gains is a great way to get your feet wet.

Now that you've listed up to 3 goals you'd like to achieve in order to grow, I'd like you to list your marginal gain for each of those things. In other words, what is a small change you can make that will help you to achieve your desired state of growth?

For example, if you have decided that you need to be more punctual for work, your marginal gain could sound something like this, "Starting from this evening, I will go to bed 30 minutes earlier each evening and wake up 30 minutes earlier."

1)

2)

3)

Now that you've thought about that marginal gain, I want to take it one step further and think about HOW you're going to achieve it.

A question for you. On average, how many people achieve their new year's resolutions?

Research suggests that on average, about 8% of people achieve their New Year's resolutions. That means that 92% of people ARE NOT achieving the change, gains, or growth that they would like to see.

I do not want you to be part of the 92% of people that fail to achieve gains, and I'm sure you do not want that either. I want you to be part of the elite 8%, and one of the keys to doing that is to create specific actions that will help you achieve your marginal gain.

Actions on HOW to achieve your goal and marginal gains can be listed out in the SMART format which stands for the following:

- Specific: The action should be clear and specific, with a well-defined outcome.

- Measurable: The action should be quantifiable, so that progress can be tracked and measured.

- Achievable: The action should be realistic and achievable, given the available resources and constraints.

- Relevant: The action should be aligned with the overall mission and values of the individual.

- Time-bound: The action should have a deadline, so that progress can be monitored and adjustments can be made as needed.

So let's go back to the ice cream scenario. If your marginal gain was to reduce the portion size of your serving to 3/4 of a cup instead of a whole cup of ice cream, how will you achieve that?

Your action might sound something like this; "Starting this evening for the rest of the week, I am going to use a 3/4 cup measuring cup to measure my ice cream servings. Once I serve and consume the 3/4 cup portion required, I will brush my teeth right after to reduce the urge to eat more. I will do this no matter where I am, at home or at a friend's or family member's house. Once the week is up, I'll re-evaluate to see if there is room for a larger reduction of my ice cream serving."

You can see that this action is:

- Specific: It includes details about the questions Who, What, Where, When, and Why.

- Measurable: It is quantifiable because it includes the metric of q 3/4 cup so that success can be tracked.

- Achievable: This isn't a drastic change, which makes it much more achievable in terms of willpower. As far as resources are concerned, as long as you can accurately measure what a 3/4 cup is, then you're good to go.

* Relevant: It is relevant because it lines up nicely with your overall goal to reduce your ice cream consumption.

* Time-bound: It is time-bound as it states when you will begin this action and how long you will continue this action before re-evaluating.

Now, I'd like you to do now is go back to the marginal gains you've designed, and write a simple SMART action that will help you to achieve it. If you can't check all of the boxes of the SMART model, that's OK, just remember that the more specific the action the better.

1)

2)

3)

In summary, you need to have a goal of a change you'd like to make, a specific marginal gain in line with that goal, and the specific action you want to take to achieve that marginal gain. The more specific the action, the better.

At this point you might be saying to yourself, "Wow! This is a lot of work!" And if you are saying that, guess what, that is discomfort speaking. But remember, once you've taken these steps and put them into action with consistency, you'll see growth happen in no time.

Next, we're going to talk about the importance of embracing failure.

2

CHAPTER TWO: EMBRACE FAILURE

ALTHOUGH FAILURE CAN BE a difficult pill to swallow, it's important to remember that it is a necessary part of growth and learning. It's not pleasant to feel demotivated and embarrassed, but these feelings can be transformed into valuable lessons if we're willing to embrace them. Failure is an opportunity to reflect, adjust and improve, ultimately leading to success in the long run.

While the fear of failure is a natural human emotion, it can have a detrimental effect on our personal and professional growth. It can keep us from taking that big leap of change. Remember this, failure is not the enemy. It's an essential part of the learning process and it can open up doors to opportunities you never thought possible. By learning to embrace failure and having the courage to take risks, you'll be able to accelerate your growth, achieve success in all areas of your life, and discover new possibilities.

Thomas Edison once said, "I have not failed. I've just found 10,000 ways that something won't work."

This quote highlights the importance of perseverance and determination in the face of failure. Edison, who is known for inventing the light bulb, is saying that failure is not the end but rather a stepping stone to success. He's saying that each failure is a new opportunity to learn and improve and that every time something doesn't work, it brings you one step closer to finding a solution that does. It's a reminder that failure should not be viewed as a setback, but rather as a valuable learning experience that can ultimately lead to success. He's trying to say that, failure is not a dead-end but a junction of new paths where you find new ways to reach your goal.

Sylvester Stallone's rise to fame is a true testament to the power of perseverance and determination. Although he now has a huge net worth and is extremely wealthy, it wasn't always rainbows and butterflies for him.

Back in the day, he was a struggling actor who faced numerous rejections, and financial difficulties, and even ended up homeless. He hit rock bottom when he was forced to sell his beloved dog for a mere $25, just to make ends meet. But, he didn't give up, instead, he found inspiration in a boxing match between Mohammed Ali and Chuck Wepner, which inspired him to write the script for the iconic film series, Rocky.

He poured his heart and soul into the script, and when he tried to sell it, he was offered a large sum of money worth $125,000, but with one condition, he couldn't star in the film. Stallone refused to let go of his dream and stood his ground, he knew that he had to be the one to bring Rocky to life. He was again offered a large sum of money worth $250,000, but he continued to stand his ground that he should be the star of the film. After much negotiation, the studio agreed, and Stallone was given the opportunity to both write and star in the film for just $35,000. The rest is history, Rocky was a huge success and went on to win numerous awards, including Best Picture and Best Directing at the Oscars, and Stallone was even nominated for Best Actor.

But Stallone's greatest victory was not the Oscar, it was buying back his beloved dog whom he had to sell for survival. It's a heartwarming tale of a man who never gave up and went on to achieve greatness despite all odds.

So what's the point? Failure is not just an uncomfortable experience, it's also a valuable one. Many successful people attribute their success to their failures, as it has taught them valuable lessons and made them more resilient. Failure allows us to learn from our mistakes, grow, and improve. Instead of fearing failure and playing it safe, we should embrace it as a necessary step toward achieving our goals.

Moreover, we must understand that failure is not a sign of inadequacy or incompetence, it is just a part of the process of achieving success. Success is full of ups and downs, and the only way to reach our destination is to keep moving forward, learn from our failures, and keep pushing ourselves. It's important to understand that failure is not a measure of our worth as human beings, it's just a temporary setback and a chance to grow. We should not let it stop us from pursuing our passions and our dreams.

So how can you push through moments of failure and come out stronger on the other side? Here are 3 very practical and effective steps that you can start using today.

1) Take Accountability: Acknowledging our mistakes and failures can feel uncomfortable and vulnerable, but it is the first step towards making things right and improving ourselves. When we take responsibility for our actions, we are not only being honest with ourselves, but we are also showing respect for others. If our failure has impacted others, it is essential that we admit our mistake, apologize, and assure them that it will not happen again. This not only demonstrates accountability but also demonstrates a willingness to make amends and improve. By owning up to our mistakes and failures, we open ourselves up to the possibility of learning and growth.

2) Analyze And Evaluate Room For Growth: When we fail, it can be hard to accept that we are not good enough - yet. But it's important to remember that failure is not a final destination, it's a stepping stone to success.

When we fail, we are given valuable feedback on what we need to improve and do differently. For example, if you are learning another language and someone is having trouble understanding what you're saying, it's a chance to reflect on what you need to change to become more understandable and communicate better in the target language.

It's important to remember that you have the power to learn from your mistakes and improve. Your failure is not a reflection of your worth as a person, it is an opportunity to grow and become better. It's not about being good enough now, it's about becoming good enough through learning and growth.

Don't shy away from failure, embrace it as an opportunity to learn, grow and improve. Remember, if you are not good enough yet, with effort, you will be.

Should you happen to fail at something in the future, ask yourself these questions:

- What actions or decisions did I make that contributed to the outcome?

- What steps can I take to prevent this type of outcome from happening again in the future?

- What is something positive that I can take away from this experience?

- How can I use what I've learned in other areas of my life?

- How is reflecting on this and using it going to help me grow?

Such questions will help you to evaluate and analyze the change needed to achieve an even better version of yourself.

3) Take Action: One of the most important things to do after learning an important life lesson is to take action. Use the lessons you learned to make positive changes in your life. This means actively applying the lessons you learned in your daily life and making them a part of who you are.

For example, if you learned a lesson about the importance of communication, make an effort to improve your communication skills and actively practice them in your relationships and interactions. Or if you learned a lesson about the importance of self-care, make a plan to incorporate self-care activities into your daily routine. Taking action is the only way to turn the lessons you've learned into real growth and progress.

Now that we've gone over 3 of the most important steps that you can take in the face of failure, let's practice.

Take a moment and think about something that you've experienced lately that didn't turn out the way you wanted it to or something you might consider a failure. Go ahead and write that down in the space below.

Next, think about and write down the answers to these questions. Feel free to write the answers in the spaces after each question.

- What actions or decisions did I make that contributed to the outcome?

- What steps can I take to prevent this type of outcome from happening again in the future?

- What is something positive that I can take away from this experience?

- How can I use what I've learned in other areas of my life?

- How is reflecting on this and using it going to help me grow?

Now that you've analyzed the answers to these questions, take the action needed to turn this into a reality. For help with that, feel free to review some of the information we talked about in chapter one about marginal gains.

Next, let's talk about the importance of actively seeking feedback.

3

— : —

CHAPTER THREE: SEEKING FEEDBACK

"Average players want to be left alone. Good players want to be coached. Great players want to be told the truth." Doc Rivers (NBA coach and player)

DOC RIVERS IS A highly successful former NBA basketball player and coach. His words suggest that the level of a player's skill and ambition is directly related to their willingness to receive feedback and criticism. Average players are content with their current abilities and do not seek out coaching or advice. Good players are eager to improve and are open to coaching. Great players, however, desire the most honest and direct feedback in order to continue pushing themselves to reach the highest level of performance.

The truth is that seeking feedback is closely related to the growth mindset because it allows individuals to gain a better understanding of their strengths and weaknesses, and to identify areas in which they can improve. People with a growth mindset believe that they can always improve, and this is an important tool for gaining the information they need to do so.

When people seek feedback, they are actively seeking out new information and perspectives that can help them to grow and develop. This can be in the form of constructive criticism, suggestions for improvement, or positive reinforcement. Additionally, people who do so are more likely to be seen as coachable and open to learning, which can lead to more opportunities for growth and development.

Seeking feedback can also help to improve performance by identifying areas where an individual is excelling and areas that need improvement, which can help to set goals and establish a plan for development. It also provides a sense of accountability, as the individual is aware that their progress is being monitored and evaluated.

So what will help you actively seek out the feedback you need to grow? Here are four steps to success.

1) Have A Purpose In Mind: Specifically identify what it is you need this feedback for. For example, maybe you're looking to improve your public speaking skills, or even more specifically, maybe you're looking to increase your eye contact with the audience as you deliver your speech. Or perhaps you want to know how to make friends easier, and more specifically, how to connect with people on an individual level the first time you're meeting them. With a purpose in mind, you'll be able to ask for the specific feedback you're looking for.

2) Smart Questions: Getting the correct guidance and feedback requires smart questioning. Take a moment to think about areas where you may need improvement or where you sense a gap and prepare open-ended questions that will help you get the information you need to fill that gap. So what are open-ended questions?

Open-ended questions require a more in-depth answer and can't simply be answered with a yes or no. Here are some examples:

- What specifically could I have/can I do differently?

- What do you think is the root cause of the issue?

- What do you see as my strengths and weaknesses in this area?

- How do you think I can improve in this area?

- What advice do you have for me to succeed in the future?

- Can you help me understand your perspective on this situation?

- What opportunities do you see for me to grow and develop in this area?

3) Ask The Right Person: When on the lookout for advice, always put the source first and foremost in your mind. Turn to people whose intentions you trust and

whose point of view is reliable. Surround yourself with individuals you interact with frequently and whose opinions you respect. Those people might include colleagues, teachers, parents, a trusted friend, a guidance counselor, a manager, or even a classmate. The point is, they should be trusted enough to give you truthful feedback.

4) Implement, Implement, Implement: To make the best use of feedback, it's crucial to reflect on what you were told and to have a plan for implementation. Start by writing down the suggestions you receive and create a step-by-step plan for putting it into action. Prioritize the changes you can make immediately and break down larger changes into manageable strategies. This is a great time to implement the theory of marginal gains as was mentioned earlier in this book.

In summary: First, have a purpose in mind by identifying what exactly you will be needing this feedback for. Second, compile some specific questions you'd like to ask for more targeted feedback. Third, choose an individual whose opinion you respect to give you honest feedback. Fourth, create a simple plan to implement the feedback.

Here is an example of how this could look in action.

Have a Purpose In Mind: My purpose is to identify areas of improvement in my presentation skills and to receive feedback to enhance them.

Compile Questions: I will ask the person giving me feedback to answer these questions specifically.

* What do you think were the strengths of my presentation?

* What specifically do you think I can improve on?

* Can you give specific examples of when I could have done better?

* How can I make my presentations more engaging and interactive for the audience?

Choose an Individual: I choose my colleague who has years of experience in public speaking and has given several successful presentations in the past.

Plan of action: I will engage in the following course of action.

* Review the feedback received from my col-

league and identify the common themes.

* Create a list of action items for improvement, for example, work on body language, use of visuals, and audience engagement.

* Schedule a mock presentation and get feedback from my colleague to assess my progress.

* Repeat the process until I am confident with my presentation skills and consistently receive positive feedback.

Now it's your turn! Please take a moment to think about something you'd like to get feedback on that will help you to grow. Once you have thought of something, complete steps 1-3 by thinking of the purpose for this feedback, questions you'd like to ask the person delivering the feedback, and the individual you feel should give you the feedback. Pause here and take a moment and write these things down.

1)

2)

3)

Once these three steps are complete, remember to take some time to write down a plan of action that will help you achieve your next level of growth.

Now let's move forward into the next phase of growth and talk about reframing limiting beliefs.

4

—:—

CHAPTER FOUR: REFRAMING BELIEFS

L IMITING BELIEFS ARE THOUGHTS or ideas that
hold you back from achieving your goals or living
the life you want. These beliefs come from a variety
of sources, including past experiences, social conditioning, cultural influences, and personal thoughts and
perceptions. For example, past experiences such as
failures, rejections, or traumatic events can lead to the
formation of limiting beliefs about one's abilities and
self-worth.

Social conditioning, including messages and beliefs,
passed down from family, peers, and society, can also
shape our limiting beliefs. Cultural influences and personal thoughts and perceptions can also contribute to
the formation of limiting beliefs. Ultimately, limiting
beliefs are a result of a combination of these factors

and can have a significant impact on an individual's behavior and decision-making.

Take the story of John as an example. John had always wanted to become a doctor. He loved learning about the human body and had a passion for helping others. However, his dreams were constantly being crushed by his limiting belief that he was not smart enough to be a doctor. This belief had been ingrained in him from a young age by his parents, who constantly told him that he wasn't cut out for such a challenging profession.

Despite his desire to become a doctor, he was haunted by the voice of his parents, telling him that he would never be able to make it in such a demanding field. He began to believe that he was indeed not smart enough, and started to focus on finding a more achievable career. He took on jobs that were less demanding, and never really pushed himself to reach his full potential.

However, as time went by, John started to feel restless. He realized that he was settling for a life that was not fulfilling and that he was not living up to his full potential. He started to question his limiting belief and began to research more about becoming a doctor. He discovered that many successful doctors had faced similar challenges and had overcome them with hard work and determination.

John made the decision to pursue his dream and enrolled in a pre-med program. He worked hard, studying long hours and asking for help when he needed it. He also started to surround himself with people who believed in him and encouraged him to reach for his dreams. Slowly, he started to break down the limiting belief that he was not smart enough and began to develop a growth mindset.

Years later, John graduated from medical school, and became a successful doctor, helping people and making a difference in their lives. He was finally living the life he had always dreamed of and was grateful for having overcome his limiting belief. He realized that the only thing that had held him back was the belief that he was not smart enough, and that anything was possible with hard work and determination.

The point of this story is that limiting beliefs can hold us back from reaching our full potential and pursuing our dreams. However, with hard work, determination, and a positive mindset, we can overcome these beliefs and achieve great things.

So what are some common limiting beliefs that we need to fight against?

Some common examples of such limiting beliefs include the following:

- "I'm not good enough."

- "I can't do it."

- "I'm not worthy of love/success/happiness."

- "I'm not smart/talented/capable enough."

- "I'll never change/improve."

- "I can't trust anyone."

- "I'm too old."

- "I'm too young."

- "I don't have enough experience."

- "I'm not smart."

Keep in mind that limiting beliefs can take many different forms and may vary from person to person and you can identify what your limiting beliefs are by looking inward at your feelings, and emotions, and by listening to the little voice in your head in a moment of challenge.

With this in mind, let's talk about a technique to conquer these beliefs called reframing. Reframing is a strategy used to adjust your mindset in order to see a situation from a different perspective. It may include reframing a problem as a challenge or looking at things from a more positive perspective.

Take the example of Sarah. According to her music teacher in school, she was musically challenged. Sarah was a young girl who had always loved music. She would hum tunes to herself as she went about her day, and would often spend hours listening to her favorite songs. However, one day in music class, her teacher told her that she was not musically inclined and would never be able to play an instrument well. Sarah was crushed. She had always dreamed of becoming a musician.

But Sarah was a determined girl. She didn't want to believe what her teacher had told her, and she refused to let that negative thought hold her back. Instead, she decided to reframe the situation. She told herself that everyone starts somewhere and that her teacher's opinion was just one person's point of view. She also realized that she was already making music, simply by humming tunes to herself. She decided to start there and began practicing her singing every day.

As Sarah grew more confident in her voice, she also picked up the guitar. She started with simple chords, and gradually learned more and more complex pieces. With each new song she learned, Sarah felt her musical skills growing. She also realized that her teacher's negative opinion was starting to fade away.

A year later, Sarah's music teacher announced a school talent show. Sarah was nervous, but she also felt excited at the prospect of showing off what she had learned. When it was her turn to perform, she took a deep breath and started to play and sing. The audience was amazed by her beautiful voice and impressive guitar skills.

After that performance, Sarah's music teacher came up to her and apologized for what she had said a year before. She told Sarah that she was amazed by her musical abilities and that she was truly a talented musician. Sarah smiled, happy that she had overcome the negative thought and reframed the situation into a positive one. She knew that she still had a long way to go, but she was confident that she would get there. And she was excited to see where her love of music would take her.

So did you notice what Sarah did? She reframed the idea that, "She could never be a great musician," and turned it into, "Everyone starts somewhere and that was just one point of view." She didn't let that notion control her world, but reframing opened up a door of possibilities.

So let's go back to the common limiting beliefs listed prior. How can we reframe these to be more helpful and productive?

- "I'm not good enough," can become, "I am worthy of growth and have the potential to improve."

- "I can't do it," can become, "I will try and will grow from the experience."

- "I'm not worthy of love/success/happiness," can become, "I am deserving of love, success, and happiness, and I will work towards it."

* "I'm not smart/talented/capable enough," can become, "I have unique strengths and abilities, and I am capable of developing new skills."

* "I'll never change/improve," can become, "I have the power to change and make positive improvements in my life."

* "I can't trust anyone," can become, "I am worthy of healthy relationships and will work towards building trust with others."

* "I'm too old," can become, "Age is just a number, and I have valuable experiences and knowledge to offer."

* "I'm too young," can become, "Youth brings new opportunities and potential for growth, and I will make the most of them."

* "I don't have enough experience," can become, "Experience comes with time and effort, and I am willing to learn and grow in my field."

* "I'm not smart enough," can become, "I'll con-

tinue learning more and more every day."

As you can see, reframing limiting beliefs opens up a door of possibilities and helps you to stay focused on growth.

What I'd like you to do now is think of 3 limiting beliefs you've had, or at least have heard of before, and reframe them into a more productive thought. Once you've done this, share your reframed beliefs with a trusted family member or friend.

1)

2)

3)

Remember, limiting beliefs are an enemy of progress, but by reframing these beliefs, your growth opportunities will increase dramatically.

CONCLUSION

I HOPE YOU'VE ENJOYED this step-by-step guide on how to cultivate a growth mindset and get the best out of yourself. Let's recap the steps we've learned in this book.

1) Embrace Discomfort. Spend some time thinking about the things you'll need to do in order to grow as an individual, even if those things feel uncomfortable. Once you've identified what those things are, spend some time thinking about which marginal gains will help you get there, and then make a simple plan to help you achieve those marginal gains.

2) Embrace Failure. Although failure can be a difficult pill to swallow, it's important to remember that it is a necessary part of growth and learning. It's not pleasant to feel demotivated and embarrassed, but

these feelings can be transformed into valuable lessons if we're willing to embrace them. Failure is an opportunity to reflect, adjust and improve, ultimately leading to success in the long run. So remember, if you do fail, take accountability, analyze and evaluate room for growth, and take action to make the necessary improvements.

3) Seek Feedback. Those who seek feedback are actively looking for new information and perspectives that can help them to grow and develop. Additionally, people who are open to feedback are more likely to be seen as coachable and open to learning, which can lead to more opportunities for growth and development. So when you do seek feedback remember to have a purpose in mind, prepare pointed questions specific to the feedback you're looking for, choose the right person to give you feedback, and implement the feedback right away.

4) Reframe Limiting Beliefs. Limiting beliefs are thoughts or ideas that hold you back from achieving your goals or living the life you want. By reframing them into a more helpful and healthier context, you'll

find yourself breaking free from thoughts and patterns that have been holding you back.

In conclusion, a growth mindset is a powerful tool for unlocking your full potential and living a life filled with growth, happiness, and success. By embracing a growth mindset, you can overcome challenges, learn from failures, and continually improve and grow. But it all starts with taking action. So, as you close this book, I encourage you to take the first step on your journey toward a growth mindset. Embrace your potential, believe in your abilities, and most importantly, take action. Your future self will thank you for it.

Remember, the power to shape your life is within you, and with a growth mindset, the possibilities are endless. So, go out there and make your dreams a reality!

ABOUT AUTHOR

Marcus Johanssen is an author, life coach, and business trainer who brings a wealth of experience to the field of personal and professional development. With a background in coaching and psychology, Marcus has helped thousands of individuals around the globe reach their fullest potential.

Over the years, he has honed his skills as a coach and consultant, becoming a sought-after expert in his field. His unique approach blends a deep understanding of human behavior and psychology with practical, actionable advice. His desire is to make difficult concepts and ideas easy to understand so they can be applied to real-life situations. This has earned him a reputation for delivering results that are both meaningful and lasting.

His expertise and passion for personal development and coaching have not only impacted the lives of his clients, but also those of his readers. Through his books, readers have the power to unlock their full potential and create the life they've always dreamed of.

Made in United States
Orlando, FL
19 July 2023

35285247R00030